Distribution, publication, and copying in any form are prohibited and subject to damages.

TEN HYPNOSES

Copying, publishing, and sharing with third parties are only permitted with the written consent of the author. Please observe the notes on copyright and usage.

Distribution, publication, and copying in any form are prohibited and subject to damages.

Copying, publishing, and sharing with third parties are only permitted with the written consent of the author. Please observe the notes on copyright and usage.

Distribution, publication, and copying in any form are prohibited and subject to damages.

Ingo Michael Simon

TEN HYPNOSES

23

TEETH GRINDING AND NIGHT CLENCHING

Copying, publishing, and sharing with third parties are only permitted with the written consent of the author. Please observe the notes on copyright and usage.

Distribution, publication, and copying in any form are prohibited and subject to damages.

© 2024 Ingo Michael Simon
All rights reserved.
Independently published
www.ingosimon.com

Important Notes for Urgent Attention:
The contents of this book are based on the practical experiences of the author with hypnosis applications and psychotherapy in a trance state. Although the author has strived for the utmost care, errors or misunderstandings in the presentation cannot be completely excluded. Therapeutic work with people and the application of hypnosis are solely the responsibility of the hypnotist. It cannot be ruled out that parts of this book may be misunderstood or that the application of a presented procedure may cause an undesirable reaction in the client. The author also assumes no co-responsibility if work with a client is carried out with reference to the statements in this book.

The Author:
Ingo Michael Simon studied psychology and education and is a hypnotherapist with practices in southwestern Germany and Switzerland. With the help of hypnosis-supported psychotherapy, he primarily treats people with persistent psychological conditions. His practice focuses on anxiety disorders, pathological compulsions, and psychosomatic illnesses. His therapeutic offerings mainly include classical and modern hypnosis applications and the dreamland therapy he developed himself.

Copying, publishing, and sharing with third parties are only permitted with the written consent of the author. Please observe the notes on copyright and usage.

Distribution, publication, and copying in any form are prohibited and subject to damages.

Notes on Copyright and Usage

Copying, publishing, and sharing with third parties is prohibited and only permitted with the written consent of the author. Please observe the following copyright and usage guidelines.

This work has been carefully crafted and created to the best of the author's knowledge and personal experience. It comprises text templates and application guidelines for professional hypnosis sessions. The author is a licensed psychotherapist with extensive experience in psychotherapy, coaching, and personal training using hypnotic techniques and methods. Nevertheless, the author and the publisher assume no liability for the accuracy of information, instructions, and advice, nor for any typographical errors. The author and publisher accept no responsibility or liability for the application of these texts and recommendations with clients or patients, nor for any potential consequences or unexpected reactions. It is expressly noted that the application of therapeutic and advisory techniques and formulations lies solely and entirely within the responsibility of the practitioner. This also applies to adherence to the boundaries of legally regulated medical and therapeutic practices. The fact that a book containing action proposals is freely available for sale does not imply that its application with clients or patients is permitted for everyone.

Copying, publishing, and sharing with third parties are only permitted with the written consent of the author. Please observe the notes on copyright and usage.

Distribution, publication, and copying in any form are prohibited and subject to damages.

Copying, publishing, and sharing with third parties are only permitted with the written consent of the author. Please observe the notes on copyright and usage.

Distribution, publication, and copying in any form are prohibited and subject to damages.

Table of Contents

Introduction 9

Hypnosis 1 11

Hypnosis 2 16

Hypnosis 3 20

Hypnosis 4 26

Hypnosis 5 31

Hypnosis 6 36

Hypnosis 7 41

Hypnosis 8 46

Hypnosis 9 52

Hypnosis 10 57

Overview of All Titles in the Series "Ten Hypnoses" 62

Copying, publishing, and sharing with third parties are only permitted with the written consent of the author. Please observe the notes on copyright and usage.

Distribution, publication, and copying in any form are prohibited and subject to damages.

Copying, publishing, and sharing with third parties are only permitted with the written consent of the author. Please observe the notes on copyright and usage.

Distribution, publication, and copying in any form are prohibited and subject to damages.

Introduction

The series "Ten Hypnoses" is very well known in Germany, Austria, and Switzerland as a collection of texts for therapeutic work and is used by numerous psychotherapeutic practices, doctors, therapists, coaches, and other helping professionals. I am pleased to now be able to offer these texts in other countries as well.

Most therapists have their own methods for inducing and deepening trance as well as for exiting trance. Therefore, I have focused on the main part of the hypnosis. The texts in this book can be integrated as the main part into any hypnosis process.

The texts in this collection use various hypnosis techniques. I will not explain these in detail, as I assume that users have the appropriate training. It is also not necessary to understand the exact structure or functioning of the different parts. The texts can simply be read aloud, and they will have their effect.

Copying, publishing, and sharing with third parties are only permitted with the written consent of the author. Please observe the notes on copyright and usage.

Decide for yourself which text best suits your client or patient at any given time. You can also combine passages from different texts. It is not about using all ten hypnoses in sequence. It is a selection of possibilities.

I want to emphasize that books cannot replace therapy. Psychotherapy or other therapeutic treatments involve much more. A careful diagnosis is the necessary basis for deciding on the use of methods, including whether hypnosis or one of my texts should be used. Even in this case, preparatory discussions, follow-up discussions during the session, and of course, a therapeutic concept for the sequence of sessions and the content approaches are essential parts of therapy. This cannot and should not be achieved with a collection of texts.

In any case, I wish you much success in your work and I am pleased if my text templates can contribute in a small way.

Ingo Michael Simon

Distribution, publication, and copying in any form are prohibited and subject to damages.

Copying, publishing, and sharing with third parties are only permitted with the written consent of the author. Please observe the notes on copyright and usage.

Hypnosis 1

Goal Setting and Will Strengthening

You know the nightly teeth grinding and clenching of the jaw in sleep ... So far, you haven't been able to control or influence it ... But you've decided to end the grinding and clenching ... You know that you need inner relaxation for this ... Relief, so you don't have to clench at all ... Often, you had to bite through in your life ... or you clenched your teeth and pulled yourself together and controlled yourself ... but you've decided to take a new path now ... Maybe it doesn't seem so easy to just stop clenching and grinding ... The idea is actually easy because you can simply imagine that you succeed ... as a fantasy ... because what is imaginable in fantasy can become reality ... Especially at night, fantasy and imagination play a big role, as they appear in dreams that process the day ... and for you, it's clear that the dream of a night without grinding and clenching should become reality ... maybe as soon as the coming night ... You are determined ...

Mental Alignment

You align your thinking entirely with letting go of the clenching and grinding ... This special and good thought now fills you completely ... You say in your thoughts ... I let go and relax my jaw muscles ... a simple thought ... maybe too simple, you think ... Can it be so simple? ... Indeed, it's often the simple thoughts that are effective ... sometimes it's just a very simple thought that led to the grinding, so a simple thought can also end the grinding ... I let go and relax my jaw muscles ... This thought becomes the thought of today ... This thought becomes the most important thought of the following days and also the most important thought of the night ... already tonight, this simple and easy thought spreads ... I let go and relax my jaw muscles ...

Somatic Alignment (Body Suggestion)

Pay attention to your body ... notice your body feeling clearly now ... feel the deep relaxation and if you think you should relax even deeper, just allow yourself to rest even more deeply and be more and more relaxed ... You can feel this calm and relaxation ... and your perception can go along your body and finally also check the jaw muscles ... You feel the relaxation in your jaw muscles, in your face, now ... You can make it very conscious, you can relax even more there ... until your entire face and the muscles of the jaw feel completely calm ... It should always feel this calm ... It should feel this calm at night, especially when you sleep ... Feel the relaxation of your jaw muscles now ... Feel the relaxation of your entire body ... Feel the calm of the night ...

Emotional Alignment (Feeling Suggestion)

You dive even deeper into your feeling and are completely there ... in the feeling of relaxation and calm ... in your inner center, you find an increasingly beautiful and gentle calm ... You find the most pleasant and calmest spot in your body ... wherever it may be ... maybe even in this moment in your face ... but maybe also in another place ... Wherever you find the most pleasant and calm spot or zone in your body, direct your attention and concentration there ... and from this spot, the deep feeling of calm now spreads throughout your entire body ... slowly moving to your head, which relaxes noticeably ... The more you manage to concentrate on the most pleasant zone of your body, the better you can also feel the relaxation spreading and enveloping your entire body ... especially letting your jaw muscles relax now ...

Behavioral Alignment

You can do even more ... While your body is now learning to provide the deepest relaxation for your head and jaw muscles, you resolve to help your organism in the evening when you go to bed ... You resolve to lightly massage your jaw muscles with the index and middle fingers of both hands, right and left ... with gentle, circular movements and thinking ... I let go and relax my jaw muscles ... This way, you can support your body and also your deep inner self ... because this way, your muscles relax even more just before falling asleep ...

Outlook and Vision

You think about how pleasant sleeping will be once you have completely let go of the clenching and grinding ... and how clearly you can feel in the morning that your jaw was completely relaxed during the night ... You can feel it ... and now you can already imagine how wonderfully relieving and freeing that will be ... especially you can imagine that you will also be internally calmer during the day, because your organism now processes stress and burdens differently ... lets go of them faster ... lets go already during the day, so you are internally calmer ... and sleep more calmly ... You can imagine it, and everything you can imagine can become reality ... Changes become reality especially quickly when you imagine the outcome ... just like now ... exactly like now ...

Summary

You align your thinking entirely with letting go of the clenching and grinding ... This special and good thought now fills you completely ... I let go and relax my jaw muscles ... You feel the relaxation in your jaw muscles, in your face, now ... You can make it very conscious, you can relax even more there ... All pleasant body sensations go to the jaw muscles and relax them ... Before falling asleep, you think this thought I let go and relax my jaw muscles ... and gently massage your jaw muscles with your fingers ...

Hypnosis 2

Goal Setting and Motivation

... You understand that it is time to change your path to end the nightly teeth grinding as quickly as possible ... Quite impressive how well you manage to fully concentrate on this goal ... on the end of teeth grinding ...

... That's why you decided to process everything that contributed to the teeth grinding in the past ... Quite impressive how well you manage to look deeply and process the causes of the teeth grinding ...

... Yes, you start today with the deep and honest processing of all connections to teeth grinding because it frees you today ... Quite impressive how well you succeed in this ...

Task for the Subconscious

... You understand that your deep inner self can help you, and that's why you chose hypnosis to end the teeth grinding and be free ... Quite impressive how well you manage to trust your deep inner self now ...

... So you now allow your deep inner self to process and resolve all tensions and aggressions deeply, because this will make you calmer inside and out, and the teeth grinding will stop by itself ... Quite impressive how well you manage to fully trust your deep inner self and feel that it actually resolves all tensions and aggressions deeply for you ... and the tensions and aggressions disappear by themselves ...

... Yes, you now allow your deep inner self to process all tensions and aggressions deeply and thus stop the tensions and aggressions ... Quite impressive how well you manage this ...

Consciousness Control

... You understand that you will reach your goal even more easily if you treat yourself with respect and love and align your thoughts constructively ... Quite impressive how well you manage to respectfully and lovingly align and control your thoughts constructively ...

... So now you resolve to think and feel with respect and love ... Yes, I trust my deep inner self because it helps me optimally at all times ... Quite impressive how well you manage to continue trusting your deep inner self and feel that it actually helps you optimally in letting go of teeth grinding ...

... Yes, you now align your thoughts with respect and love to fully trust your deep inner self and fully support the inner processing ... You now align your thoughts with respect and love ... Quite impressive how well you manage this ...

Processing in the Subconscious

... Your deep inner self understands that there is an inner working and struggling that has led to the nightly clenching ... Your deep inner self knows all causes and connections, all unresolved and suppressed emotions that led to this attempt to get through ... Quite impressive how well your deep inner self manages to recognize and understand all this ...

... Therefore, your deep inner self takes over the task of resolving and processing these connections for you from now on and then letting go ... Quite impressive how quickly your deep inner self can accomplish this task ... Quite impressive how well you work hand in hand with your deep inner self ...

... Yes, your deep inner self is already processing all suppressed emotions in this minute, allowing them and accepting them, because this dissolves the struggle ... this dissolves the tension, and you feel inner peace and calm again ... Quite impressive how well you manage to feel inner peace already now ...

Outlook

... You understand that today is a day of true transformation, liberation, and constructive change ... Quite impressive how well you manage to embrace this change ...

... That's why you continue to trust in the support of your deep inner self, which helps you today and continues to help ... Quite impressive how well you manage to trust your deep inner self in your waking life as well ...

... Yes, you trust your deep inner self absolutely ... for the end of the nightly clenching and teeth grinding and for true inner peace ... Quite impressive how quickly the end of teeth grinding is possible ...

Hypnosis 3

Anchor Technique

As an anchor (or trigger), we refer to a stimulus that should create a certain feeling or evoke a particular thought. It is a signal perceived by the client, which then triggers an internal process. The established anchor then replaces the suggestion. In everyday life, a client can trigger a desired state or create it without a trance state using an anchor. Numerous stimuli can be used as anchors/triggers. I work with the following options, which I also use in the series "Ten Hypnoses": Physical anchors (closing the hand, pressing the ball of the thumb ...), Visual anchors (symbols, word cards ...), Acoustic anchors (signal sounds like mobile phone ringing, melodies ...), Olfactory anchors (essential oils ...), Haptic anchors (smooth stones, talismans ...). I also distinguish between perihypnotic and posthypnotic anchors. Perihypnotic anchors are primarily used during hypnosis by the therapist to set up the anchor and then trigger it repeatedly as a supplement to suggestions and visualizations. Posthypnotic anchors are set up for the time after the session so that the client can help themselves with them.

Preparation of the Anchor Technique

You want to sleep peacefully, without any clenching or grinding ... You have often thought about what it would be like to wake up in the morning and feel your jaw muscles loose and relaxed ... as relaxed as now ... and your teeth are so light that you don't even feel them ... because your teeth can rest at night too ... During the day they work, just like you ... while eating and chewing they are required, but at night the teeth have nothing more to do ... absolutely nothing to do ... You have internally set yourself up to find deep rest and relaxation and also feel it in the muscles of your face ... just like now, because now you are relaxed and also your face is relaxed ... and if you think the muscles of your face should become even looser, just let them go ... if you think your jaw muscles can relax even more, just let them go ... and everything becomes even quieter ... but there's more ... You need an anchor ... an anchor is a tool that ensures that your jaw muscles remain calm and relaxed even when you sleep ... maybe you wonder how that works ... There are many ways to set up an anchor ... You can use an acoustic anchor ... which means a sound can help you ... a sound that reminds you even in your sleep to stay loose and relaxed ... and you certainly want to know how that works ... So let's get started ...

Creating the Desired Emotional State

Relaxation is important now because your anchor works better the more relaxed you are when we set it up ... Feel your body now and check how you can best relax now ... first the feet ... Let them become calm and if you think you should move them briefly or change their position to really be relaxed, then do so ... and relax your feet ... now the legs ... Let them become calm and if you think you should move them briefly or change their position to really be relaxed, then do so ... and relax your legs ... Now it's the turn of the abdomen ... relax your abdomen ... let it become calm with a deep breath, to then really be relaxed when exhaling ... Your abdomen relaxes ... Then we move to the back ... Let it become calm and if you think you should move briefly or change your position to really be relaxed, then do so ... and your back relaxes ... Now we move to the arms ... Let them become calm and if you think you should move them briefly or change their position to really be relaxed, then do so ... and relax your arms ... Next, we move to the head ... Pay attention to the skin of your face ... especially the jaw muscles ... Let them become calm and if you think you should move your lower jaw briefly to really be relaxed, then do so ... and your whole face relaxes ... Everything becomes calm in you ... good ... it works excellently ...

Setting the Anchor

Now, in this beautiful relaxation, all sounds around you are unimportant ... The sounds of everyday life are far away and fade ... but one sound is with you ... the sound of your breath ... You hear the airflow through your nose, in and out ... You hear this gentle wind of your own breath ... and you hear it even in your sleep, just as we hear all sounds in our sleep, but they don't disturb us ... but you hear your breath best because it is very close ... it comes from you ... Focus entirely on the sound of your breath and feel the relaxation in your face at the same time ... Now follow the movements of your lower jaw ... Let it be completely loose, so that the teeth of the upper and lower jaw do not touch ... and feel how your lower jaw relaxes further when exhaling and with closed lips opens a bit more ... Consciously hear your breath now when exhaling and feel how your lower jaw becomes looser ... becomes looser and looser ... The sound of your breath becomes the signal of loosening ... The more you focus on hearing your breath, the looser your jaw muscles become ... the more relaxed your lower jaw becomes ... Hear your breath and feel the calm and relaxation now ... it works excellently at this moment ... and your body remembers it ... Hear your breath and feel the relaxation of your lower jaw ... [Wait ten seconds] ... Hear your breath and feel the relaxation of your cheeks ... [Wait ten seconds] ... Hear your breath and feel the calm in your face ... [Wait ten seconds] ... good ... very good ... it works ...

Consolidation (Posthypnotic Suggestion)

Your body has already understood and learned ... When you lie in bed and want to fall asleep, you naturally pay attention to your breath ... A part of you hears your breath and immediately remembers that this is the signal for relaxation and your cheek muscles relax ... When falling asleep, you always hear your breath, which loosens your jaw muscles ... even in sleep, a part of you hears your breath, which loosens your jaw muscles ... so your face remains relaxed all night long ... so your jaw muscles remain relaxed all night long ... every night relaxed ...

Hypnosis 4

Preparation and Will Strengthening

You want to end the clenching and grinding at night ... You couldn't control it so far; your body just clenched while you slept ... but today you can change it because your body follows your thoughts ... Strenuous thoughts at night made you clench ... Thoughts of relaxation help you let go of your jaw muscles and relax from now on ... You set your thoughts on a quiet sleep ... and it's quite impressive how well you manage and how quickly you can set your thoughts on this today ... You succeed today ... you succeed ...

Distancing Active Thoughts

Imagine you are sitting in a cinema ... An old cinema, as cinemas used to look ... with thick, soft chairs, covered in velvet ... very soft chairs ... Make yourself comfortable in a velvet-covered chair. You are all alone in this cinema. The entire hall is empty and it is quiet, very, very quiet ... Look around a bit in your cinema hall ... The floor is velvet-soft ... A very soft carpet ... Maybe a dark red ... a beautiful, very dark red ... The walls are covered with colored fabric ... Red and green ... red and green ... And from the ceiling hangs a huge chandelier, with many light bulbs and countless crystals ... It glows just enough for you to see everything well ... Make yourself very comfortable in your chair, make yourself comfortable in your soft chair ... On the walls of the cinema hang small lanterns. Two or three on each side, right and left ... In them burn small violet gas flames ... The screen far ahead is covered by a thick, heavy curtain ... A dark, heavy curtain covers the screen in this beautiful cinema ... It gets darker and darker ... The light is dimmed and it gets darker and darker ... And at the same time, you can let it become more and more comfortable and calmer within you ...

Presentation of the Affirmation

The curtain slowly opens, the long, heavy, dark curtain slides slowly aside ... The curtain opens more and more ... It gets darker and darker, quieter and quieter ... The curtain opens more and more ... The quiet hum of the projector is heard, the intro begins ... Up front on the screen is a number ... a ten ... And as the intro runs, numbers run backwards, from ten to zero. I count with you, and with each number I mention, you can sink deeper, with each single number I mention ... ten ... nine ... eight ... seven ... six ... five ... four ... three ... two ... one ... the movie is about to start ... it's about to begin ... it can start now ... zero ... now it starts ... now it begins ... And up front on the screen, in big, bold letters, it says:

I let go of all worries and problems at night for a liberating and restful sleep.

... [Read the affirmation slowly and a bit louder than the previous text to emphasize it. Then pause for about 30 seconds before continuing to read.] ...

Impact and Deepening of the Affirmation

Let the affirmation sink deep ... take it into your inner self and let it unfold its effect ... Allow yourself now calm and mindfulness ... Calm and mindfulness ... and feel how your jaw muscles loosen in this moment ... because now you succeed in letting go of the problems and worries of the day ... and everything you can experience and achieve in a state of pleasant trance, you can also experience and achieve in your waking life ... if it corresponds to your own inner goals ... and you have this goal of letting go ... of relaxing your jaw muscles at night ... to sleep calmly and pleasantly ... without grinding or clenching ... to wake up in the morning with a relaxed jaw ... with relaxed facial muscles ... Maybe you can already feel the relaxation of your jaw muscles spreading and flowing through your deep feelings ... or you will feel it in a few minutes when the affirmation unfolds even more strongly ... because it will ... It unfolds and becomes stronger until it has become your stable belief ... your new attitude of inner relaxation at night ... your inner relaxation while sleeping ... You end the grinding with your deep convinced attitude ...

Repetition and Integration of the Affirmation

Deep within you, these words work, which you read on the cinema screen and can look at again and take in once more ...

I let go of all worries and problems at night for a liberating and restful sleep.

... allow yourself now a moment of calm, without having to think or do anything ... Just be there and breathe in and out ... with wide and deep breaths ... because with the flow of your breath, the effect of the words flows deeper into your inner self ...

Consolidation (Posthypnotic Suggestion)

You've done it ... and every day you can repeat the affirmation when you go to sleep ... and as soon as you lie down, you remember the words of relaxation, and your jaw muscles relax deeply ... As soon as you lie down to sleep, your jaw muscles relax very deeply ...

Hypnosis 5

Goal Setting and Preparation

You have the firm intention to end the night clenching and grinding ... You want it to stop ... Maybe you've tried several things and set your thoughts on letting go at night, but it hasn't worked properly yet ... But you have the absolute will to give your teeth and jaw muscles rest at night ... you understand that the clenching had reasons, so it was normal for your body to clench tightly at night ... Maybe you thought it was a sign of too much effort and an expression of inner tension that couldn't fully disappear even in sleep ... and that was certainly one of the reasons for the night clenching ... So if you can relax ... sustainably relax, your body doesn't need the clenching anymore ... Today you are here so that your body gives your teeth rest at night and leaves your jaw muscles relaxed ... completely relaxed ...

Perspective Change

Imagine you were a wolf ... and the people of your everyday life, with whom you have confrontations or conflicts, were also wolves ... just as a fantasy, as an idea ... Imagine that powerful people or systems or organizations were powerful, strong wolves ... Colleagues or employees of authorities ... Lawyers or bailiffs ... or just the people you perceive as threats in your life ... Imagine them all as wolves ... These wolves scared you ... Maybe you often felt smaller or weaker than them in your waking life ... or you had a queasy feeling in your stomach when you met them ... from this sometimes a suppressed aggression arose, maybe often without you noticing it ... or you controlled yourself ... Maybe you sometimes wanted to defend yourself ... would have liked to do it with words of defense and said what you think and want ... but it wasn't possible ... Maybe you sometimes wanted to use your fangs and defend yourself ... like a wolf who can fend off attacks and opponents with his sharp teeth ... But you pulled yourself together, often swallowed the anger, and bit it into yourself at night ... to hold back ... Without biting, you couldn't defend yourself, and so the whole burden often remained within you ... only at night did your body bite, which suppressed it during the day ... symbolically biting for the restraint during the day ... You imagine the many wolves of your life ... maybe there aren't that many ... maybe only a few who are particularly dangerous, as you learned to stop biting ... and started to bite into yourself ...

Re-evaluation of Own Experiences

Let your thoughts and memories awaken, and a time comes to mind when you grinded or clenched particularly strongly at night ... Imagine the situation now again and imagine you actually had the fangs of a wolf and were in a wolf pack ... and now imagine very clearly how you clenched your teeth in this situation ... Maybe you could have defended yourself against what really bothered or strained you ... even and especially if it were internal things ... maybe memories or feelings you fought with ... because, in reality, you didn't fight but prevented yourself from fighting ... hid your fangs ... without teeth, no wolf can defend himself ... Remember this situation and stand beside yourself ... Watch yourself clenching your teeth in silence more and more ... how you made yourself a wolf without teeth without noticing it ... Maybe then you can already see that you often would have liked to defend yourself instead of clenching your teeth ... Imagine many wolves standing before you with sharp teeth, and you keep your mouth closed to be a very nice wolf ... hoping to be left alone ... There they are, the wolves of humiliation ... wolves of fear ... wolves of inner conflict ... wolves of hopelessness ... and such wolves that only you know ... Their teeth are and remain dangerous ...

Action Change

In your fantasy, in your thoughts, you change this picture now ... So imagine you could immediately stop clenching your teeth ... and imagine opening your mouth to show your teeth ... in your fantasy, this is quite easy and happens very quickly ... and deep inside you, it also happens just as quickly ... You show your teeth ... you open your mouth and show your teeth ... teeth of anger ... teeth of determination ... teeth of your inner strength ... like a wolf, you show your teeth so you don't have to clench at all ... to show that you can and will defend yourself if you are pressured ... in everyday life, you will defend yourself with words ... with determination and decisions ... here in the fantasy of the wolf pack, you do it with your teeth ... showing teeth instead of clenching them ... showing teeth instead of clenching them ... You imagine it that way ... You see yourself ... see yourself showing your teeth ... and at the same time, you see how the wolves become more cautious ... cautious wolves of humiliation ... cautious wolves of fear ... cautious wolves of inner conflict ... cautious wolves of hopelessness ... and such cautious wolves that only you know ... The inner wolves that threatened you so often become more restrained, and you gain strength and power ...

Consolidation (Posthypnotic Suggestion)

You now feel the inner calm and relaxation ... You feel and you know that you can fend off the wolves inside you ... You feel and you know that you can show your teeth ... and exactly this helps you to sleep better at night because in relaxation arises the strength to show your teeth during the day ... Your body helps you with relaxed sleep ... from now on ...

Hypnosis 6

Goal Setting and Preparation

You want to end the night clenching and grinding ... if you could command your body, it would already be over ... but you can do something much better because you can actually get your body to stop clenching and grinding at night ... It is an expression of the unresolved ... Anger that has not yet been settled ... Problems that are not yet solved cling to you and make you clench at night ... You couldn't control it so far ... but today you can ... today you can do something to end this strain at night ... can limit the burden that expresses itself there to the day ... because during the day, you can do something and act, not in sleep ... so it is important and right to postpone burdens you feel when falling asleep or that are simply unnoticed there ... Maybe you noticed that postponing actually means putting it on the day ... That's what you do today ... You put the problems with all their challenges on the days ... and find peace and looseness at night ...

Setting up the Place of Encounter

Deep inside you, there is a place of encounter ... a place where you can meet yourself ... it lies within you, and you find it by now concentrating on the feeling of your body ... Imagine you can dive into your inner center ... being in the middle of your body ... and there you let it become darker and darker because you dive deeper and deeper into your own feelings ... Everything becomes dark and black because the impressions outside become unimportant ... the perception of the space becomes more and more insignificant ... You let yourself sink down into a deep darkness and calm ... It becomes quieter and quieter within you ... and more and more comfortable and calmer ... and suddenly, you see a small light inside you that quickly grows larger ... You are at the place of inner encounter ... You meet yourself ... it is like in a room where you stand opposite yourself ...

Meeting with the Inner Helper

Deep inside you, you stand opposite yourself ... a calm and experienced part of you ... because that is also a part of you ... Calm and experience ... You are surrounded by light, and you feel light ... much lighter than before ... and opposite you stands this image of yourself ... You are there to help yourself ... like a friend who comes to your aid ... who is here now to help you in this situation ... a friend who is here now to help you find rest and relaxation at night ... who can take the burdens from you without ignoring them ... This helper stands before you ... Your helper ... [Please adjust to the client's gender] ... greets you with a heartfelt hug ... with a warm feeling that you can feel in your body now if you pay close attention to your body feeling ... You feel this warmth and feel the connection to yourself ... to this helper within you ...

Confrontation and Clarification

You think about everything that made you grind your teeth at night ... what led to you clenching so tightly at night ... You surely know some causes and reasons ... others remained hidden from you so far ... So you ask your helper what they know about it ... and this part of you looks at you lovingly ... sends you thoughts and feelings now or even speaks to you ... You now learn something new about the reasons for clenching ... Just listen and feel what they tell you inside now ... [Now give about 30 seconds time] ... Just accept what your inner image tells you because it is a message from you to you ... from deep within you, from your inner center ... whatever you received or think, let it be there because it is an important part of the nightly strain ... even if you couldn't hear or feel anything yet, don't know what your inner self wants to tell you today, you can stay calm and relaxed ... because all answers are within you ... they lie in your feeling and are there even without words ... can soon show themselves in your consciousness and come into your thoughts ... your inner helper is here to truly help you ... with answers, but also with actions ... this part of you that looks like your image carries a small valuable casket with them ... a small treasure chest ... Your helper opens the chest, and you look inside ... it is empty ... Then your helper places their hand on your forehead, and it feels as if all worries and problems are taken from you at this moment ... It is as if this inner part of you takes over all the worries and problems to free you in your thoughts ... and then your helper places these worries and problems as small balls in the chest ... All the worries and problems, the unresolved things that made you clench at night, you now place in an inner treasure chest ... There your inner helper keeps these challenges for you ... finds new solutions and approaches while you sleep in peace ... and during the day, you get the treasure chest back with these new solutions and approaches ...

Consolidation (Posthypnotic Suggestion)

Your inner helper closes the chest and says goodbye ... So it should happen every evening ... So it should always be when you want to sleep ... just before falling asleep, you automatically meet yourself, deep in your feeling ... and a part of you takes and keeps all worries and problems over the night ... develops solutions in peace while you sleep in complete peace and relaxation ... only after getting up in the morning do you get the treasure chest back with challenges and solutions ... just like today ... exactly like today ...

Hypnosis 7

Goal Setting and Preparation

Today you want to let go of the tensions that made you clench and grind in the past ... You know what it's like to grind or clench your teeth at night without intending to ... Actually, you wanted to relax ... You want to relax now and every day, so you can sleep peacefully ... Grasp during the day and relax at night, that's your goal ... your declared will ... and nothing is more important now than achieving this goal ... but not with stubbornness ... Stubbornness has only led to clenching so far ... your organism has gotten used to it ... but now is the time to relearn ... your organism learns a change today ... Let go in sleep and grasp in wakefulness ... Let go in sleep and grasp in wakefulness, that's what it comes down to ...

Somato-emotional Change

So, let's go ... Thoughts were sometimes strenuous even in sleep without you noticing it ... but at night in sleep, you cannot solve difficulties, you cannot grasp them ... that is not necessary either because at night when you sleep, you need recovery ... you can gather strength to grasp during the day ... Grasp instead of clenching ... Grasp instead of clenching ... You can do that ... in fact, you don't clench during the day ... not even when you say you are biting through ... It's a figure of speech because you don't have to clench ... but your body clenches at night ... clenches through or clenches teeth because there is the thought of persevering and enduring ... So today we first want to teach your body to behave differently so that you can experience restful sleep again ... and can sleep restfully every night ...

... Focus your mindfulness now on your cheek muscles ... Feel into it ... Feel how it feels ... Maybe your cheek muscles are already relaxed now ... or you can still feel a certain tension or movement even now in the calm of trance ... That's perfectly fine ... the better you can perceive the change in a moment ... Now place the fingertips of your index fingers on the cheek muscles on both sides ... Then clench your teeth briefly because then you feel where the muscles push out the most ... Place your fingertips there ... [Wait until the client has positioned their fingers correctly] ... good ... That's right and works best ...

... Now massage these two muscles with gentle pressure of your fingers and with light, circular movements so that the muscles relax further ... [Please give about 30 seconds time] ... good ... Now let the fingers rest quietly on the cheek muscles and feel the relaxation with your fingertips because you can feel it with your fingertips ... because any tension that might still be there goes from the jaw muscles into the fingers ... This way, the cheek muscles relax deeper and deeper ... and you also come to more inner calm ...

... With light palpation, you can feel the relaxation of the cheek muscles ... can experience and check that at this moment the tension indeed fades and your jaw joints become loose ... become looser and looser ... as loose as the tongue ... Maybe you noticed that the tongue doesn't tense, no matter what happens ... even when the teeth clenched or even ground, the tongue was loose and relaxed ... and so now the cheek muscles also relax and any tension that might still be there is massaged away by the fingertips ... This way, your body sets itself to grasp during the day and let go at night ... grasp during the day and let go at night ... Your body shows you that it works as soon as you can feel the relaxation of the cheek muscles clearly ... For this, you just need to feel your cheek muscles with your fingertips and, if you want, massage a bit ... then you can feel the relaxation clearly ... Focus on your fingertips ... The better you manage to feel the contact of your fingertips with your cheek muscles, the faster they relax ... it happens automatically ... and there's more because your body has already relearned ... Maybe you already noticed the inner change of your body ... or you can perceive it in a few moments ...

... Now place your hands back beside your body ... and feel that your cheek muscles are indeed relaxed and remain relaxed ... You can feel it ... Now your cheek muscles are truly relaxed ... because your body has replaced the previous connection between strenuous thoughts and clenching with letting go at night and grasping during the day ... You can feel that your tongue is completely relaxed and calm ... and just as relaxed and calm are now your jaw muscles ... completely relaxed and calm ... and so it remains at night ...

Consolidation (Posthypnotic Suggestion)

Maybe you wonder how to best keep it that way ... and maybe it surprises you to hear that your body has already relearned and will ensure that your cheek muscles remain relaxed at night ... Your body helps you ... and you can help your body ... Just place your fingertips on your cheek muscles on both sides shortly before sleeping and notice how the tension in your muscles decreases ... with light massaging you make the signal to your body even clearer ... and immediately your cheek muscles relax and become as loose and relaxed as your tongue ...

Hypnosis 8

Ideomotor Responses

Ideomotor responses refer to the phenomenon where our body follows our feelings and thoughts with movements. In everyday life, this following is shown as posture, muscle tension, and movement patterns of a person, naturally changing with the mood and thoughts. In trance, ideomotor signals can be used to obtain information that the client cannot actively communicate. The subconscious can, for example, answer questions with an agreed finger signal. Of course, ideomotor responses can also be used suggestively, for example with arm levitations and catalepsies. An ideomotor approach strengthens trust in hypnosis and in one's own ability to change, thus promoting therapy.

Setting Up Finger Signals

Dear subconscious of ... [client's name] ... with the index finger, you greeted me and showed your willingness to cooperate ... thank you for that ... The index finger should therefore be the finger with which we can communicate because nothing should happen that you don't truly want deep inside ... You know that only you can change everything ... that only you can deeply end the grinding and clenching ... and for that, I offer you my help ... You can move the index finger whenever you want to say YES ... As soon as you are ready to find another way with my help today, a way that has nothing to do with grinding and clenching, please show me a signal with the YES finger ... [Wait until the signal occurs clearly, if necessary, ask again] ... You are already ready ... good, then let's get started ... You can now free yourself from the grinding and clenching ... It is very easy ... because there is a reason for the grinding and clenching ...

Replacing the Disruptive Behavior (Reframing)

Subconscious of ... [client's name] ... I know there is a reason for the nightly clenching and grinding ... You are trying to communicate and show something ... But what you are trying to show cannot be understood ... The mind tries, but it hasn't succeeded so far ... But I know you can act differently ... In the infinite variety of your possibilities, you can, subconscious of ... [client's name] ... find a new way, a way that has nothing to do with clenching and grinding ... Everything that happens has meaning, even the clenching and grinding, but it burdens you more than it helps ... So you can replace it ... What you want to communicate to the mind, you can do in another, gentle way because you are much more creative than clenching and grinding ... So look in the infinite variety of your creativity for another behavior that is pleasant and therefore much more suitable than clenching and grinding ... If you imagine that it can succeed, then you can also imagine that it is helpful to end the clenching and grinding, because then the mind has much more freedom and strength to take good care of you ... So find a new way, and I know you can ... Find a way here and today without clenching and grinding ... just for you ... just for you ... You, subconscious of ... [client's name] ... can end the annoying clenching and grinding today ... because you find a new and pleasant way ...

Decide deep inside, subconscious of ... [client's name] ... the mind doesn't have to know ... whatever you do ... Just delete the clenching and grinding once and for all and replace it with a pleasant reaction of the body ... a pleasant reaction that lets you sleep well at night ... and as soon as you have done that, move the YES finger ... As soon as you have managed to turn off the clenching and grinding and replace it with pleasant and helpful actions, show me the YES finger ...

[Wait patiently because the finger will move and send a reliable message about an actual inner change. My experience shows that the subconscious of people is very reliable and indeed establishes lasting changes if it confirms so. In return, the client should regularly consciously encounter themselves in everyday life with mindfulness. For example, in a weekly meditation or mindfulness exercise, listen to yourself. This keeps the initiated change stable in the long term. If the subconscious does not move the YES finger, gently encourage again ... I know you can do it, and as soon as you have managed to end the clenching and grinding, show me the YES finger ...]

There is the signal ... thank you, you did it ... You replaced the clenching and grinding ... found a new and better way for yourself ... That's very good because it lets you sleep much better and also be fresher and stronger during the day ... This way, you succeed in forming a unity of thoughts and feelings ... being one with yourself ... very good ...

Stabilizing the New

Now it is time to stabilize your new way so that you can let go of the clenching and grinding forever ... Test your new way, your new idea ... Imagine you are sleeping without clenching and grinding, just as you have just decided ... Look at it and optimize your new way until it becomes completely good for you without clenching and grinding ... Create your new sleep program without clenching and grinding and show me with the YES finger as soon as you are done ... [Wait until the finger moves] ... good ... You did it ... You freed yourself from clenching and grinding ... freed yourself forever ...

Releasing the Ideomotor Responses

You have taken an important step and now everything will be different ... I thank your subconscious for this support ... You can now give back control of the right hand to consciousness ... Consciousness and subconscious flow into each other and become one ... You can now let go of all images and fantasies inside and feel good in your whole body ... Allow yourself another moment of calm and trust that you have indeed freed yourself from clenching and grinding ...

[Try to be patient if the signals come hesitantly. Ideomotor signals are reliable signs, similar to kinesiological muscle tests. The brief reframing presented here is very effective in practice when ideomotor signals are given as confirmation. If communication with finger signals is difficult, deepen the trance with simple suggestions in between. More detailed work with reframings can be found in my book "Reframing in Trance".]

Hypnosis 9

Preparation

You have a goal, a clear goal ... You want to stop grinding and clenching your teeth at night ... It's as if you bite through every night ... or just clench your teeth and hold on ... But you want to end it ... sometimes thoughts and worries stick, making it difficult to let go at night ... But it can also be easy to break this connection ... Today we are working on exactly that ... teaching your body to rest at night ... and be relaxed ... to keep the jaw muscles and the skin of the face relaxed or to relax them again and again ... So you set yourself up for this goal ... with your thoughts and with your strength ... good ... That's how it can succeed ...

Presupposition

You often tried to fight against the cramps and strenuous thoughts ... Today it should be different because you want to break the connection between strenuous thoughts and clenching ... so problems and worries can be there, but you let go ... All topics can be, but you let your cheekbones and jaw muscles relax ... Today it comes down to perceiving something else ... your hands ... and the more you succeed in concentrating on the feeling in your hands, the faster the tensions in the face dissolve ... The more you succeed today in feeling your hands, the faster your body learns to stay relaxed at night ... to keep your jaw muscles relaxed and relax them even more ... Feel your hands for a moment now ... [Wait ten seconds] ... good ...

Current State and Goal Setting

And now remember what it's about ... So far, the clenching and grinding at night bothers you ... But this is how it should be from now on ...

Complete relaxation of the jaw muscles and cheek muscles

with calm and relaxation in the face

... [When speaking the goal setting, feel free to place your palm on the client's solar plexus and then remove it. It is not required, but it helps a lot because the goal setting is thus "anchored". Of course, you can also incorporate energetic techniques into the hypnosis. Be careful not to repeat the goal.] ...

Building the Emotionally Balancing Frame

Now let go of your thoughts and direct your mindfulness to something else ... your hands ... Let your hands lie loosely beside your body and try to feel how they feel ... Maybe they both feel similar ... or one is a bit warmer than the other ... and maybe it's not so easy to feel both at the same time, but you try ... possibly it's easier to feel the right hand first and then the left hand ... but over time you succeed in perceiving both simultaneously and fully concentrating on the feeling ... because over time, both will match in their feeling ... Pay attention to the feeling in your hands and simply wish them to feel the same ... equally warm ... as if both hands were connected ...

... Your thoughts are now only about your relaxed hands ... they lie beside your body, and you can perceive them ... everything else is now irrelevant ... and it feels good to deal with just one perception for once ... You don't need to interpret it; it doesn't matter why your hands feel as they do now ... it's just important to really feel them ... and that succeeds now ... at this very moment ... It succeeds very easily and playfully, to focus on your hands and keep them calm ... and if you still feel a slight tension in your hands, just let go again ... because now it only matters that your hands relax ... and you can feel that now ... Check if both hands feel the same ... and if that is not the case now, it will happen in a few moments ...

... Now slowly move your mindfulness from your hands to your arms ... over the forearms and upper arms to the shoulders ... and from there to your face ... and to your lower jaw ... to the cheekbones and the jaw muscles ... and feel that they are indeed relaxed ... good ... You can feel it ... Everything is calm and relaxed ...

Dissolving the Energetic Frame

Now let your thoughts wander back and forth ... Now nothing is important anymore, and you don't have to pay attention to anything ... Your body has already integrated this relaxation ... The connection between problem thoughts and clenching and grinding has already changed ... because you are more balanced internally ... and your body reflects that through loose jaw muscles ... through relaxed jaw muscles ... This way, you can come to rest and relax every day if you want ... simply by concentrating on your hands ... on both at the same time ... because then the same thing happens as today ... You relax very deeply ... and even at night when you sleep, your jaw muscles remain relaxed ... completely relaxed in sleep ...

Hypnosis 10

Arriving in the Land of Dreams

Today you can undertake a special journey ... a journey that leads you into and through a foreign land that is also a very familiar land ... the land of dreams ... It lies somewhere inside you ... in your imagination ... in your own world of ideas, where you can think of anything ... You can create it yourself or let yourself be surprised by inner images, ideas, or thoughts ... but it will always be very familiar because it arises deep in your feelings ... The land of dreams is always a reflection of your moods and feelings ... an expression of your feelings ... You reach there with the power of your thoughts ... are already there because a part of us is always in our own dreams and visions ... You are in the land of dreams and just let the images arise ... images of a beautiful and unique land ...

Confrontation, Clarification, and Creative Reorientation

You stand on a meadow under the open sky and look up ... The sky is covered with gray clouds ... They hang like pressing thoughts over you ... You look ahead, and in front of you lies a huge pile of gray stones ... and as if by itself, you start to climb up, to climb the stone heap ... You step over the rubble and rocks step by step upwards ... On your way up, you think of the many obstacles that existed or exist in your life ... it comes to mind how difficult it often was to step over the stones that lay in your way ... some were maybe just there, and you didn't even know where they came from ... kept going and bit through ... others were perhaps put or rolled in your way, but you couldn't prevent that ... kept going and bit through ... You only know it that way, always continuing and biting through ... but sometimes it was too much, and you found no way out anymore ... You know what it's like when you approached solving difficult tasks with determination ... often you had no other choice than to be determined ... so it happened that you even tried to bite through in your sleep ... or more precisely, your body displayed what your thoughts did when falling asleep ... biting through ... and in sleep, the thoughts continued to circle ... You bit through, and also your teeth clenched ...

... You keep climbing upwards ... climb the mountain of stones ... bite through on this strenuous path ... but in the land of dreams, there are no strenuous paths ... here everything is much easier than in the waking everyday life ... because here you can change everything ... with the power of your thoughts, you can change your paths ... with the power of your feelings, you can change your paths ... So you stop ... You stay in place and feel the need to take a break ... Be it ever so easy in the land of dreams, you want to rest ... You want to find stillness and calm to recharge ... so you go down, climb back down from the rubble heap ... and reach the meadow ...

... You want to rest ... later you can still climb the hill ... You look around for a quiet and comfortable place ... You discover a thick old tree with wide branches ... You go to the tree, and the warming sunrays touch your body ... You look up ... The sky is bright and clear ... Meanwhile, all the gray clouds have moved on ... You didn't notice it, but now you can see it ... maybe they will come back and soon bring bad weather, but for today the clouds are gone ... Now the sky is bright and clear, and the sun is shining ... You lie down under the protective branches of the tree ... Its long branches and dense foliage cast a pleasant shadow ... You find a comfortable mattress or a soft blanket under the tree

... and lie down on it to lie very comfortably and sleep a bit ... It is warm, and you slowly become tired ... You look once more at the mountain, the hill of rubble and stones ... at the many obstacles that lay in your way ... but now you want to sleep ... You need a break ... And slowly your eyes close ... You become more and more tired and just let yourself fall ... trust the soft ground of the dreamland, which is the ground of your own soul ... and there you can only lie softly ... soft and safe ... soft and safe ...

... Then you feel that every tension in you dissolves, and everything becomes quieter ... a warm summer wind gently blows over your face and loosens your jaw muscles ... and a fine humming reaches your ear ... You open your eyes again ... they have become heavy and sluggish, but you want to see where this humming comes from ... There you see small, nimble elves, no bigger than a finger of your hand ... They fly like hummingbirds around you and carry small pots with a balm with them ... a fragrant and relaxing balm, which they rub on your cheeks with their small hands ... You feel the relaxation that arises ... and full of trust that the elves do the best for you and help you relax and let go, you close your eyes ... You feel the balm on your skin and the relaxation of your cheek muscles ... Now you don't have to bite through anything because now is the time just for you ... the time of your recovery that you can find in sleep ... Here in the land of dreams, sleep is always restful sleep ... and what is possible here is also possible in the waking everyday life ... just a moment later ...

Mindfulness and Self-Fidelity

Then you sleep very deeply and dream a beautiful relaxing dream of the time when there will be no more biting through in your waking everyday life ... because you never have to bite through again ... because everything finds and results, even when you have to strive and solve many problems ... You end the clenching in the land of dreams ... and slowly you awaken again in the land of dreams and feel the relaxation in your face ... You open your eyes and look at the mountain of stones, which has suddenly disappeared ... you can only see some gray sand ... only some gray sand ... Here this is possible, but much more happens in the land of dreams than just a dream or a fantasy ... Deep inside, everything changes, and you can sleep relaxed at night ... because the land of dreams is in you and has always been there ... I just tell you about it ...

Distribution, publication, and copying in any form are prohibited and subject to damages.

Overview of All Titles in the Series "Ten Hypnoses"

Volume 1: Smoking Cessation
Volume 2: Anxiety and Restlessness
Volume 3: Burnout
Volume 4: Reducing Overweight
Volume 5: Coping with the Past
Volume 6: Suicidal Thoughts and Attempts
Volume 7: Psycho-Oncology
Volume 8: Obsessions and Tics
Volume 9: Self-Confidence and Decision-Making
Volume 10: Grief Work
Volume 11: Psychosomatics
Volume 12: Chronic Pain
Volume 13: Depressive Thoughts
Volume 14: Panic Attacks
Volume 15: Domestic Violence, Victim Support
Volume 16: Post-Traumatic Stress
Volume 17: Exam Anxiety and Stage Fright
Volume 18: Anti-Violence Training, Offender Support
Volume 19: Addiction Tendencies
Volume 20: Social Phobia and Fear of Contact
Volume 21: Nail Biting
Volume 22: Self-Awareness and Self-Love
Volume 23: Teeth Grinding and Night Clenching
Volume 24: Feelings of Guilt
Volume 25: Fear in Crowds
Volume 26: Fear of Flying, Aviophobia
Volume 27: Fear in Enclosed Spaces, Claustrophobia
Volume 28: Tinnitus, Ear Noises
Volume 29: Fear of Heights
Volume 30: Neurodermatitis

Copying, publishing, and sharing with third parties are only permitted with the written consent of the author. Please observe the notes on copyright and usage.

Volume 31: Finding Inner Balance
Volume 32: Overcoming Loneliness
Volume 33: Fear of Illness, Hypochondria
Volume 34: Anticipatory Anxiety, Fear of Fear
Volume 35: Jealousy in Relationships
Volume 36: Driving Anxiety
Volume 37: New Start after Separation
Volume 38: Fear of Injections
Volume 39: Heart Anxiety Neurosis
Volume 40: Overcoming Resentment and Anger
Volume 41: Resolving Blockages and Positive Thinking
Volume 42: Stress Reduction, Stress Management
Volume 43: Body Relaxation
Volume 44: Deep Relaxation
Volume 45: Fear of the Dark
Volume 46: Falling Asleep and Staying Asleep
Volume 47: Compulsive Buying
Volume 48: Restless Legs Syndrome
Volume 49: Bulimia
Volume 50: Anorexia
Volume 51: Overcoming Nightmares
Volume 52: Imagined Deformity
Volume 53: Overcoming Distrust, Finding Trust
Volume 54: Processing Failures
Volume 55: Humiliation, Emotional Hurt
Volume 56: Distressing Compassion, Vicarious Suffering
Volume 57: Self-Forgiveness
Volume 58: Self-Awareness, Self-Confidence
Volume 59: Saying No
Volume 60: Assertiveness
Volume 61: Setting Boundaries and Self-Assertion
Volume 62: Decision-Making Ability

Volume 63: Success Orientation
Volume 64: Ruminating, Circular Thinking
Volume 65: Accepting Pregnancy
Volume 66: Birth Preparation
Volume 67: Spiritual Opening
Volume 68: Joy of Life and Inner Lightness
Volume 69: Patience and Inner Peace
Volume 70: Fibromyalgia and Rheumatism
Volume 71: Irritable Bowel Syndrome, Crohn's Disease
Volume 72: Fear of Nausea, Emetophobia
Volume 73: Stuttering and Cluttering, Speech Flow Disorders
Volume 74: Concentration and Knowledge Anchoring
Volume 75: Vitality and Spontaneity
Volume 76: Searching for Meaning and Finding Goals
Volume 77: Life Crises, Life Events
Volume 78: Workaholism, Goal Obsession
Volume 79: Helper Syndrome, Helpless Helpers
Volume 80: Medication Abuse
Volume 81: Gambling Addiction
Volume 82: Internet Addiction, Smartphone Addiction
Volume 83: Hoarding Disorder, Compulsive Collecting
Volume 84: Conspiracy Thoughts, Overvalued Ideas
Volume 85: Fear of Operations and Treatments
Volume 86: Fear of Aging
Volume 87: Travel Anxiety
Volume 88: Anxiety When Urinating, Paruresis
Volume 89: Fear of Intimacy and Togetherness
Volume 90: Fear of Blushing
Volume 91: Coming Out in Homosexuality
Volume 92: Charisma Training
Volume 93: Migraines and Chronic Headaches
Volume 94: Overcoming Allergies, Bronchial Asthma

Volume 95: Normalizing Blood Pressure
Volume 96: Compulsive Perfectionism
Volume 97: Sports Hypnosis, Motivation
Volume 98: Sports Hypnosis, Performance Enhancement
Volume 99: Determination and Focus
Volume 100: Encountering the Inner Child
Volume 101: Cravings, Binge Eating
Volume 102: Stimulating Metabolism
Volume 103: Bipolar Mood Swings
Volume 104: Borderline, Identity Crises
Volume 105: Hypomania, Euphoria, Mania
Volume 106: Restlessness, Agitation
Volume 107: Nervous Breakdown
Volume 108: Adjustment Disorders
Volume 109: Self-Alienation, Depersonalization
Volume 110: Ending Self-Pity
Volume 111: Primary Gain of Illness
Volume 112: Secondary Gain of Illness
Volume 113: Bullying, Victim Support
Volume 114: Letting Go of Envy and Jealousy
Volume 115: Fear of Spiders, Arachnophobia
Volume 116: Fear of Dogs or Cats
Volume 117: Fear of Strangers, Xenophobia
Volume 118: Excessive Worries, Generalized Anxiety
Volume 119: Strengthening Sense of Responsibility
Volume 120: Unrequited Love, Heartache
Volume 121: Work-Life Balance
Volume 122: Letting Go of Unattainable Goals
Volume 123: Allowing and Accepting Help
Volume 124: Letting Go of Adult Children
Volume 125: Tourette Syndrome
Volume 126: Life Changes and New Starts

Volume 127: Accepting Life in a Wheelchair
Volume 128: Understanding and Overcoming Homesickness
Volume 129: Understanding and Overcoming Wanderlust
Volume 130: Dizziness, Meniere's Disease
Volume 131: Overcoming Aggression
Volume 132: Cutting and Self-Harm
Volume 133: Hair Pulling, Trichotillomania
Volume 134: Postpartum Depression
Volume 135: For Relatives of Dementia Patients
Volume 136: Self-Harm, Artificial Disorders
Volume 137: Activating Self-Healing Powers
Volume 138: Preventing Depression Relapse
Volume 139: Reactive Psychoses, Follow-Up
Volume 140: Obsessive Thoughts and Impulses
Volume 141: Compulsive Checking
Volume 142: Compulsive Counting, Symmetry Obsession
Volume 143: Compulsive Washing, Cleanliness Obsession
Volume 144: Compulsive Questioning
Volume 145: Dissociative Paralysis
Volume 146: Phantom Pain
Volume 147: Overcoming Complaining
Volume 148: Hay Fever, Pollen Allergy
Volume 149: Sexual Abuse, Victim Support
Volume 150: Standing Strong Against Sexism, #metoo
Volume 151: Binge Eating
Volume 152: Overcoming Thoughts of Revenge
Volume 153: Detachment from the Aggressor, Stockholm Syndrome
Volume 154: Courage to Separate
Volume 155: Chronic Fatigue, Exhaustion
Volume 156: Fear of the Future, Existential Anxiety
Volume 157: Excessive Worry About Children
Volume 158: Fear of Failure

Volume 159: Ending Distrust and Control
Volume 160: Dejection, Dysphoria
Volume 161: Boreout, Chronic Boredom
Volume 162: Bipolar Disorders, Relapse Prevention
Volume 163: Mania, Relapse Prevention
Volume 164: Nihilism, Feelings of Worthlessness
Volume 165: Thumb Sucking
Volume 166: Being Brave
Volume 167: Being Proud
Volume 168: Overcoming Shyness
Volume 169: Being Able to Delegate Responsibility
Volume 170: Being Able to Show Emotions
Volume 171: Letting Go of Guilt, Victim Support
Volume 172: Processing Guilt, Offender Support
Volume 173: Mood Swings, Cyclothymia
Volume 174: Lack of Drive, Vital Sadness
Volume 175: Hearing Voices with Reality Reference
Volume 176: Confident Communication
Volume 177: Standing Up for Oneself
Volume 178: Taking New Paths
Volume 179: Confident Job Application
Volume 180: No Longer Being Taken Advantage Of
Volume 181: End of Submissiveness
Volume 182: Depressive Numbness
Volume 183: Mood Drops, Affective Incontinence
Volume 184: Mood Instability
Volume 185: Somatoform Disorders
Volume 186: Stomach Ulcer, Psychosomatic
Volume 187: Accepting Amputation
Volume 188: Overcoming and Letting Go of Hatred
Volume 189: Ending Accusations
Volume 190: Allowing Tears, Being Able to Cry

Volume 191: Finding and Sorting Repressed Feelings
Volume 192: Somatoform Pain
Volume 193: Living Autonomously
Volume 194: Anhedonia, Joylessness
Volume 195: Persistent Sadness
Volume 196: Obesity, Food Addiction
Volume 197: Parents of Abused Children
Volume 198: Letting Go and Letting Be
Volume 199: Childhood Sexual Abuse
Volume 200: Fear of Loss

www.ingramcontent.com/pod-product-compliance
Lightning Source LLC
Chambersburg PA
CBHW030459220526

45464CB00006B/2580